SUZANNE BYRD

ADHD: Unleashing the Superpower Within

Copyright © 2025 by Suzanne Byrd

All rights reserved. No part of this publication may be reproduced, stored or transmitted in any form or by any means, electronic, mechanical, photocopying, recording, scanning, or otherwise without written permission from the publisher. It is illegal to copy this book, post it to a website, or distribute it by any other means without permission.

First edition

*This book was professionally typeset on Reedsy.
Find out more at reedsy.com*

Contents

1. Introduction to ADHD as a Superpower — 1
2. Reframing ADHD: Strengths at a Glance — 6
3. The Science Behind ADHD — 11
4. Creativity Unleashed: The Artistic Mind of ADHD — 16
5. The Hyperfocus Advantage — 22
6. Resilience and Grit: Navigating Challenges — 27
7. Social Skills and Innovation: The Connector's Edge — 33
8. Finding Your Passion: The Key to Motivation — 38
9. Tools for Transformation: Practical Strategies for... — 44
10. Education: Changing the Narrative in Schools — 50
11. In the Workplace: Transforming Career Paths — 56
12. Conclusion: Celebrating the Superpower Within — 62

1

Introduction to ADHD as a Superpower

In a world that often equates traditional success with predictability and sameness, Attention Deficit Hyperactivity Disorder (ADHD) has long been viewed through a narrow lens of dysfunction. For many, ADHD conjures images of distracted individuals flitting from one shiny object to another, struggling to navigate the demands of modern life. But what if this perception was fundamentally flawed? What if, instead of merely dwelling on the challenges, we could unveil the hidden potential beneath the surface—a superpower waiting to be acknowledged and unleashed?

This book, *"ADHD: Unleashing the Superpower Within,"* is a passionate exploration into the intricacies of ADHD, revealing a vibrant landscape of creativity, resilience, and innovation that often goes unnoticed in the shadows of traditional narratives. In the pages that follow, we will delve deeper into the unique attributes of individuals with ADHD, supported by personal anecdotes, case studies, and scientific resources that converge on one central thesis: ADHD is not a disorder to be "cured," but a distinctive trait to be embraced.

The Traditional Perception of ADHD

The historical treatment of ADHD has often seemed punitive. Children labeled with this condition are frequently subjected to extra scrutiny in environments designed for order and compliance, where adherence to norms is favored over divergence from them. The societal narrative presents ADHD not only as a hurdle but as a heavy burden that individuals must carry through life—a veritable mark of failure that signifies inadequacy in the face of norms. The stigmatization of ADHD can be debilitating, creating barriers that hinder acceptance and understanding.

But there is an alternative narrative—one that sings the praises of what it means to think differently. To illustrate this, let me share the story of Maya, a 28-year-old graphic designer whose journey encapsulates the transformation of challenges into strengths. Maya's childhood was anything but smooth; her teachers deemed her "disruptive," often reprimanding her for daydreaming or fidgeting during lessons. The label of ADHD felt like a heavy weight around her neck, impacting her self-worth as she transitioned into adolescence.

In her darkest moments, Maya felt suffocated by societal expectations; she believed herself to be inherently flawed. That was until she began to embrace her unique processing style, realizing that her inability to focus on boring tasks was counterbalanced by her capacity to dive deeply into subjects that fascinated her. It was this epiphany—this acceptance of her ADHD—that marked the turning point in her life. By harnessing her hyperfocus during creative peaks, Maya won several design competitions, ultimately becoming a sought-after talent in her field. Her story serves as a reminder that what is seen as a deficit can, in fact, pave the way for people like Maya to ignite their creativity and reshape their careers.

Emerging Insights and Research

Research into ADHD is evolving, challenging outdated conceptions and highlighting the unique attributes found in those with the condition. A groundbreaking study published in the *Journal of Attention Disorders* demonstrated that individuals living with ADHD often exhibit heightened levels of creativity and unconventional thinking, key attributes essential for innovation across various domains. Notably, the cognitive patterns associated with ADHD can lead to remarkable lateral thinking, allowing individuals to connect disparate ideas and formulate solutions that others might overlook.

Consider the case of an entrepreneur named Raj. Raj was once viewed as the "class clown" in school, rarely able to sit still or concentrate during lectures. However, upon entering the business world, he discovered that his propensity for risk-taking and outside-the-box thinking was precisely what his budding tech start-up needed. While conventional business acumen typically favors meticulous planning and a measured approach, Raj's improvisational style and spontaneity led his company to pursue groundbreaking ventures that ultimately doubled their market share. Raj learned, as many individuals with ADHD do, that the very qualities that seemed impractical as a child could flourish in the entrepreneurial landscape, reshaping his identity and success.

As we navigate through this book, we will take a closer look at these strengths and the science behind them, encouraging readers to redefine their understanding of ADHD. We will delve into important discussions about how ADHD contributes not just challenges but extraordinary abilities such as creativity, resilience, and social skills—characteristics often considered essential to modern innovation and collaboration.

Transforming Perceptions

The journey toward re-framing ADHD into a celebrated characteristic requires a collective shift in understanding. It is an evolution that begins at the grassroots level—within families, schools, workplaces, and communities. The stories of Maya and Raj are not isolated; they are part of a larger tapestry showcasing countless individuals who have channeled the supposed limitations of ADHD into extraordinary achievements. This book aims to serve as a beacon of hope and transformation, illustrating how ADHD—often deemed a hindrance—can become a superpower.

Ultimately, by asking ourselves to look beyond traditional perceptions and serving as advocates for this evolution, we encourage others to recognize the diverse strengths within themselves and the individuals around them. Through acceptance, we forge connections that allow us to leverage these unique traits for growth and success.

As we journey through each chapter, we will reinforce the belief that ADHD is a multifaceted lens through which creativity and innovation can flourish. It's a call to arms—an invitation to embrace not just the diversity of thought that ADHD brings but also our shared humanity that connects us all.

The path to viewing ADHD as a superpower begins here. Are you ready to break free from the constraints of conventional

thinking? Let us embark on this exploration together, celebrating the rich tapestry that is the ADHD experience and the superpower within us all.

2

Reframing ADHD: Strengths at a Glance

ADHD, Attention-Deficit/Hyperactivity Disorder, has long been boxed into a narrative of deficits — a disorder characterized by inattentiveness, impulsivity, and hyperactivity. However, as emerging research begins to unveil, ADHD traits can also be the wellspring of extraordinary capabilities. Recognizing and nurturing these strengths can transform the lives of individuals with ADHD, leading them to flourish in creative, innovative, and high-demand environments.

Central to understanding ADHD as a superpower is identifying its core traits: creativity, hyperfocus, risk-taking, and resilience. These are not mere quirks but rather a unique blend of characteristics that can propel individuals toward monumental achievements. With these ideas in mind, let's delve deeper into the advantages afforded by ADHD traits, illustrated through impactful anecdotes and compelling case studies.

Creativity: The Catalytic Force

Consider Jenna, a graphic designer whose award-winning work has graced the covers of magazines worldwide. From the outset of her career, Jenna was often dismissed during group projects, labeled as "distracted" or "unfocused." But what her colleagues didn't realize was that while she appeared to flit from one idea to the next, her wandering mind was actually crafting a rich tapestry of concepts that would later unfold into intricate designs.

Jenna's signature style — a fusion of eclectic colors and bold patterns — was born from her ability to see connections between seemingly disparate ideas. Armed with ADHD, Jenna learned to harness her creativity by embracing her continuous stream of ideas. Each potential design became a thread for a larger narrative, allowing her to produce work that resonated deeply with audiences. It was during a particularly challenging project, with a tight deadline looming, that Jenna unlocked her hyperfocus — an intense period of concentrated effort that allowed her to invest her creativity in a way that yielded stunning results under pressure.

Research corroborates Jenna's experience, with many successful entrepreneurs and artists possessing ADHD. In a recent survey conducted by the Journal of Creative Behavior, over 60% of creative professionals identified as having ADHD. They attributed their ability to innovate, think outside the box, and drive their projects to successful conclusions to the unique cognitive processes associated with their ADHD.

Risk-Taking: Embracing the Unconventional

Furthermore, individuals with ADHD often exhibit a propensity for risk-taking. While this trait can lead to impulsive decisions, when channeled effectively, it can also result in groundbreaking innovation. Take the case of an entrepreneur named Alex, who turned down a conventional corporate career to launch a fintech startup. Alex understood the importance of challenging norms and the power of calculated risks — two attributes intimately linked to the ADHD experience.

During a pivotal moment in his business journey, Alex faced a crucial decision: invest the majority of his earnings into a revolutionary app or play it safe. Guided by his ADHD-enhanced intuition, he opted for the bold move. The app not only changed the way small businesses handled their finances, but also won numerous industry awards. Alex's story exemplifies how risk-taking isn't simply a byproduct of impulsivity; it's often the catalyst for transformative success.

The Hyperfocus Advantage

Hyperfocus, a period of intense concentration that can be both a boon and a challenge for those with ADHD, is a trait deserving of special mention. This phenomenon allowed Matt, a software developer, to revolutionize the way his team approached coding. During a particularly daunting project, Matt disappeared into his coding workspace, coding for nearly 72 hours straight, fueled by the excitement of problem-solving and creativity. It was within this hyper-focused state that he identified flaws in their initial software design, reimagining an entirely new model that not only resolved existing bugs but advanced the product's capabilities beyond the original vision.

To capitalize on hyperfocus, Matt implemented strategies to create "focus blocks" in his schedule, setting specific times dedicated exclusively to coding. He created an environment free from distractions and utilized tools like timers and task lists to maintain clarity about short-term goals, helping him navigate tasks with greater ease.

Studies highlight the mixed nature of hyperfocus, revealing

that it drastically increases productivity levels in those who can effectively harness it. A systematic review published in the journal *Attention Disorders* concluded that hyperfocus, when appropriately directed, facilitates enhanced problem-solving and innovation, leading to successful outcomes in both academic and workplace contexts.

Resilience: The Gift of Endurance

Living with ADHD often cultivates resilience — a vital skill in navigating both personal and professional challenges. Michelle, a professional athlete, faced numerous hurdles stemming from her ADHD, including difficulty with concentration and organization. However, these challenges became her stepping stones to triumph. Michelle recounted a pivotal moment in her career: during a major competition, she felt overwhelmed by the distractions of the crowd. Instead of succumbing to anxiety, Michelle leaned into her training and utilized specific mental techniques, born from her necessity to cope with ADHD, to regain focus.

By developing a unique set of coping strategies — mindfulness exercises combined with creative visualization techniques — she not only excelled at her sport but became a mentor for others facing similar challenges. Her success is substantiated by a study in the *Journal of Sports Psychology*, which found that individuals with ADHD often develop greater resilience through adversity, enabling them to confront challenges more fearlessly.

Conclusion: Turning Challenges into Opportunities

Reframing ADHD traits from mere challenges to remarkable superpowers is not just an exercise in semantics; it opens the door to a world of possibilities. From creativity that fuels innovation to risk-taking that drives monumental shifts in industries, the attributes associated with ADHD are pivotal in today's fast-paced, ever-evolving landscape.

As we lean into this framework of understanding, it becomes clear that substituting traditional notions of ADHD as a deficit with a recognition of its potential as a source of strength can change lives. Jenna, Alex, Matt, and Michelle, along with countless others, serve as guiding lights, illustrating how embracing ADHD — with its rich tapestry of traits — can unleash a unique brand of power capable of transforming not just individual lives, but entire industries.

For those navigating the world with ADHD, embracing these strengths may require a shift in self-perception, but it is one that can unlock a lifetime of opportunities. The stories of successful individuals point to a wider narrative: that ADHD, when reframed and harnessed, is less of a disorder and more of a superpower just waiting to be unleashed. It's time to celebrate and amplify the strengths within us, paving the way for a future where individuals with ADHD are recognized for their extraordinary contributions and innovative capabilities.

3

The Science Behind ADHD

In a world eager to label the behaviors and traits of individuals, many with ADHD found themselves under a microscopic lens, often viewed through a narrow lens of deficits and failures. However, as we delve deeper into the complexities of ADHD, it becomes increasingly clear that the neurological underpinnings of this condition are not merely indicative of a disorder, but rather the scaffolding from which exceptional talents can emerge. This chapter serves as an exploration of ADHD from a scientific perspective, shedding light on the unique brain differences that contribute to the superpower qualities of those diagnosed with this condition.

A Neurologist's Perspective

Meet Dr. David Reyes, a neuroscientist with ADHD. Growing up, David faced the pervasive struggle of distraction and impulsivity typical of many individuals with ADHD. However, rather than allowing these traits to stifle his ambition, David harnessed his unique brain wiring to become one of the leading researchers in the field. In his journey, he discovered that outgoing thoughts and quirky ideas are not just by-products of his ADHD; they were key to his innovative research methodologies.

During a recent podcast interview, David shared, "There was a point where I realized that my brain worked differently, but that wasn't a hindrance—it was a gift. I was able to view problems from angles that my peers didn't even consider." David referenced a pivotal study in which he and his team discovered that individuals with ADHD exhibited increased activity in multiple areas of the prefrontal cortex, responsible for attention and decision-making, compared to those without ADHD. This hyperactive brain function translated into enhanced problem-solving capabilities—often finding pathways to innovation that others could not.

To appreciate the full impact of these neurological differences, it's essential first to understand what we mean by ADHD. Attention Deficit Hyperactivity Disorder is characterized by patterns of inattention, hyperactivity, and impulsivity that can affect daily functioning and development. Traditional views emphasized deficiencies, leading to the oversimplified narrative of ADHD as a mere 'disorder'—something to be managed or eradicated. Emerging research, however, is reshaping that narrative, reframing ADHD as a cluster of diverse traits that can lead to remarkable abilities when properly nurtured.

Breaking Down the Neurological Make-up of ADHD

The brain of an individual with ADHD is a magnificent puzzle filled with intriguing twists and turns. Advanced imaging studies reveal differences in the sizes and structures of certain brain regions, particularly the frontal lobe and the basal ganglia. For instance, the frontal lobe, which governs executive functions such as impulse control and organization, is often found to be less active in individuals with ADHD. Yet, paradoxically, at times of hyperfocus—a hallmark trait of ADHD—this same area lights up remarkably, showcasing the unique potential buried within.

Furthermore, the neurotransmitters dopamine and norepinephrine play significant roles in how individuals with ADHD experience the world. Low levels of dopamine are believed to underlie the difficulties with motivation and focus. However, when engaging in highly stimulating or interest-driven activities, many with ADHD find themselves in a state of profound focus, pushing boundaries and uncovering innovative solutions. This contrasts starkly with neurotypical brains, which may not experience the same rush of creativity and inspiration.

The Breakthroughs and Studies

In a study conducted at the University of California, researchers gathered a group of individuals diagnosed with ADHD and subjected them to a series of problem-solving tasks. What they discovered was astonishing: participants with ADHD not only solved problems more creatively but were also adept at thinking outside the box. Their unique neurological wiring, characterized by increased connectivity and flexibility in brain networks, allowed them to approach challenges from unorthodox angles. This begged the question: could ADHD actually provide an edge in creative and innovative thinking?

In another landmark study published in the Journal of Cognitive Neuroscience, researchers explored the nuanced experience of distraction among individuals with ADHD. Rather than a mere deficit in focus, the study illustrated how distractions could spark new thoughts and ideas. Participants reported that interruptions often led to significant breakthroughs in their tasks. This phenomenon could be considered a reframe of what is typically deemed as a lack of attention; instead, it's an illustration of how diversely wired neural pathways can result in spontaneous creativity.

Real-World Applications of ADHD Traits

The scientific backing for these unique attributes of ADHD opens doors for individuals across various fields. Take, for example, the world of technology—a field ripe for innovation. Individuals with ADHD have become some of the leading figures in tech start-ups, where rapid iteration and creative problem-solving are key to success. One renowned entrepreneur, Sarah Kim, who was diagnosed with ADHD at a young age, credits her ability to think divergently as a significant factor in her tech company's meteoric rise. In interviews, she often highlights how her unconventional approaches have led to breakthrough features that competitors had never considered. "My brain is like a web of connections—sometimes chaotic, but often yielding unexpected solutions," Sarah remarked during a TED Talk that celebrated neurodiversity in entrepreneurship.

Also worth noting is the rich tapestry of creativity found in the arts. Renowned creatives—from musicians to visual artists—have often spoken of their ADHD experiences as vessels for their artistic expression. One can think of famous figures like Vincent van Gogh and his posthumous recognition for a bright, loaded emotional palette, or how author J.K. Rowling broke down genres with her fantastical world-building in the Harry Potter series—both renowned individuals believed to have exhibited traits associated with ADHD.

Conclusion: Embracing the Neurodiverse Brain

The science behind ADHD not only allows for a richer understanding of the brain but also lays the groundwork for practical frameworks within society to embrace its intricacies. Assessments focusing on competencies rather than deficiencies can lead to enhanced perceptions of individuals with ADHD, transforming cultural narratives and opening doors to new paths of achievement.

The journey from being perceived as disruptive to understanding innate superpowers is monumental. Embracing these brain differences can equip individuals with ADHD not just for personal success, but also empower them to leave lasting impacts on their communities. In the following chapters, we will explore the unique attributes of creativity and hyperfocus as gifts that can be cultivated and harnessed to unleash the true potential of individuals with ADHD—a community of innovators, creators, and leaders waiting to emerge into the spotlight.

4

Creativity Unleashed: The Artistic Mind of ADHD

An Artistic Perspective

In our world that celebrates creativity, those with ADHD often possess an innate ability to think divergently, forming connections that others might overlook. This chapter explores the profound link between ADHD and creativity, offering a lens through which we can appreciate the unique artistic expressions of individuals living with this condition. We're delving into the rhythms of creative minds whose vibrant imagination not only enriches the arts but also transforms personal challenges into vibrant masterpieces.

The Frequency of Inspiration

Take, for instance, the story of Laura, a musician whose melodies have captivated audiences worldwide. From a young age, Laura struggled with traditional learning environments. The flurry of thoughts and stimuli often overwhelmed her in classrooms where silence was the norm. Instead, she found solace in music—a space where her hyperactive mind could roam free. With ADHD, she frequently experienced fluctuations in her focus, which could be a double-edged sword. Yet, when she latched onto a musical idea, her ability to hyperfocus transformed that single concept into a symphony of sound.

"I can spend hours just lost in a chord progression or working on a lyric. When I'm in that zone, it's like nothing else exists," Laura recounted. This wave of creativity didn't just yield songs; it brought her global recognition and accolades, highlighting how ADHD fueled her artistic voice. Laura's experience reflects a broader trend found among many artists diagnosed with ADHD, demonstrating that their unconventional thought patterns can lead to groundbreaking work.

The Connections Between ADHD and Creativity

Research substantiates the connection between ADHD and creativity, particularly in the realms of the arts. A study published in the *Journal of Creative Behavior* noted that individuals with ADHD often exhibit the traits of divergent thinking—an essential element of creativity. Divergent thinking allows for multiple solutions to a problem, leading to innovative ideas rather than conventional approaches. When traditional norms do not bind creative individuals, they can push boundaries and explore novel concepts.

Another renowned artist, Vincent van Gogh, is a classic example. His vibrant brush strokes and emotive use of color mirrored his tumultuous mental state, often attributed to his undiagnosed ADHD. Van Gogh's struggle with impulsivity and restlessness became the driving force behind expressive pieces that are now regarded as masterpieces. This historical connection illustrates a pattern: those navigating ADHD frequently experience a unique lens of perception that catalyzes artistic expression.

Beyond the Canvas: A Deeper Exploration

To delve deeper, let's examine contemporary case studies within the artistic realm. One prominent figure is Sir Anthony Hopkins, the esteemed actor and composer who received an ADHD diagnosis later in life. Known for his dynamic character portrayals—from the chilling Hannibal Lecter to the whimsical Odin—Hopkins attributes his ability to fully immerse himself in diverse roles to his ADHD. He once articulated, "It's a gift. It allows me to experiment freely, unencumbered by societal norms or fear of judgment."

This sentiment resonates within the field as studies indicate that ADHD individuals often possess heightened emotional sensitivity, granting them the ability to draw deeply from personal experiences, emotions, and ideas. This sensitivity in the encapsulation of emotion cultivates profound connections with audiences, allowing for an authentic expression that transcends mere performance.

The Role of Environment in Artistic Flourishing

The environments that nurture creativity among those with ADHD play a critical role. Understanding the necessary conditions to support this creativity can lead to positive outcomes. For Laura, having her own studio space—where she could immerse herself in sound without interruption—was vital. It was in this creative sanctuary that remarkable ideas blossomed. Similarly, the expansive landscapes of nature inspired writers like J.K. Rowling, whose ADHD-driven experiences spurred the creation of beloved worlds filled with fantastical adventures.

Historically, many successful individuals with ADHD, including business magnates like Richard Branson, have cited the importance of flexible environments conducive to unleashing creativity. Empowered by their unique traits, these individuals have often paved pathways where traditional routes did not exist, fostering industries and paving the way for innovative endeavors.

Patterns of Resilience and Ingenuity

In a broader sense, the creative instincts of individuals with ADHD are often intertwined with resilience and ingenuity. This connection affords artists a unique perspective when faced with obstacles. The histories of those within creative fields reveal a consistent theme of overcoming failures and rejections, much like the improvisational nature of jazz music.

Consider the literature of author Jack Kerouac, whose spontaneous prose style reshaped American literature. Kerouac's own battles with ADHD resulted in a lurching, evolving narrative style that mimics the fluidity of thought he experienced. His journey underscores how barriers faced due to ADHD can birth an innovative art form, exemplifying the resplendence of creativity in juxtaposition with struggle.

Innovations in Artistic Collaboration

The creative mind of individuals with ADHD also emphasizes the power of collaboration. Artists often come together to enhance their vision, meeting diverse ideas that can be reinvigorated by ADHD's versatility. Collaborations that harness neurodiversity yield art where myriad perspectives contribute to a multifaceted creation.

Consider the collaboration between artists that led to the famed Broadway production *Hamilton*, where inclusion and leveraging individual talents alongside personal challenges became the bedrock of innovation. A multitude of voices, including those with ADHD, fueled a narrative and creation process that broke traditional boundaries, showcasing the magnetic power of creativity amidst challenge.

Final Thoughts: Embracing the Superpower of Creativity

As we explore the artistic minds of individuals with ADHD, it becomes evident that their inherent creativity is a superpower waiting to be unleashed. The stories of Laura, Vincent van Gogh, and Anthony Hopkins illustrate a broader movement where creative pursuits catalyze not just personal expression, but cultural revolutions.

Unlocking this creativity involves creating nurturing ecosystems where individuals with ADHD can thrive—environments that recognize their unique contributions to the world. Encouraging the fusion of creativity and the art of living with ADHD propels society toward embracing neurodiversity, highlighting the importance of alternative forms of genius.

As we conclude this chapter, remember that those with ADHD carry within them the seeds of innovation, inspiration, and artistry. Rather than viewing ADHD through the lens of limitation, we must celebrate creativity as a mighty superpower, one that leads to extraordinary feats and enriches our shared human experience. Let this journey inspire you to recognize and cultivate the creative forces around you, fostering spaces where imagination can run wild and thrive.

5

The Hyperfocus Advantage

In the ever-evolving dialogue surrounding Attention-Deficit/Hyperactivity Disorder (ADHD), one of its most compelling and paradoxically beneficial features is hyperfocus. While ADHD is often characterized by distractibility and impulsivity, hyperfocus emerges as a powerful trait, enabling individuals to deeply engage in tasks that ignite their passions. This chapter will delve into the nature of hyperfocus, its advantages, and how it can be harnessed effectively. Through a mixture of anecdotes and case studies, we will explore how individuals have transformed their lives and industries by embracing this unique neurological feature.

To understand hyperfocus, we must first recognize its definition. Hyperfocus is a state of intense concentration on a particular task or idea, often to the exclusion of everything else. When in this zone, individuals with ADHD can work for hours, wholly immersed in their endeavor, often achieving remarkable results. Unlike the fleeting attention spans that characterize ADHD, hyperfocus can feel almost meditative, leading to a sense of flow that many creators and high achievers crave.

Anecdote: The Programmer's Journey

Consider the story of Alex, a talented programmer who discovered his knack for hyperfocus during college. Tasked with a difficult coding assignment, he found himself under immense pressure to deliver results. As the deadline loomed, distractions seemed to evaporate, and everything around him faded into the background. He entered a state of hyperfocus, diving deeply into the complexities of his project.

"Time disappeared," Alex recalls. "In that space, I was invincible. I coded and coded, algorithms making sense in new ways. I had no idea how long I had been working until I looked up. Hours had passed, and I had finished what was supposed to take weeks."

The outcome was not just a successful project but also the genesis of a revolutionary app that streamlined online communications for developers. Alex's hyperfocus allowed him to tap into his creativity and problem-solving abilities simultaneously, producing something extraordinary. This experience not only boosted his confidence but also set him on a trajectory toward a successful career in tech.

Understanding Hyperfocus: The Neuroscience Behind It

The phenomenon of hyperfocus is rooted in the neurological differences often found in individuals with ADHD. Studies suggest that the brain's reward system is highly sensitive in those with ADHD, with dopamine levels playing a significant role. When engaged in activities that are enjoyable or stimulating, the brain releases a surge of dopamine, resulting in laser-sharp focus. This biological mechanism can propel individuals into hyperfocus, where they work at a heightened level of productivity.

Recent research has highlighted how the prefrontal cortex and other areas of the brain responsible for executive function are activated during periods of hyperfocus. This unusual pattern of brain activity can bypass typical attention deficits, allowing for exceptional output in specific circumstances. Understanding this underlying science not only legitimizes hyperfocus as a natural advantage for those with ADHD but also underscores the potential benefits when individuals learn to channel it effectively.

Case Study: Innovators Who Embrace Hyperfocus

A compelling case study comes from the world of entrepreneurship. Many successful business innovators have thrived by recognizing and utilizing their hyperfocus. Take, for instance, the story of a tech entrepreneur named Sarah, who built an acclaimed digital marketing agency. Diagnosed with ADHD in childhood, Sarah faced numerous challenges in academia and the corporate world. However, she learned to recognize the moments when hyperfocus kicked in—typically when facing a new project or client challenge.

By establishing her own business, Sarah was able to curate an environment conducive to her hyperfocus. "In my own company, I was able to structure my day around my strengths. The moment I get excited about an idea or strategy, I dive deep. I can work for days on end without losing steam," she said, emphasizing the importance of a flexible work environment.

Sarah's ability to harness hyperfocus not only led to the successful acquisition of multiple high-profile clients but also fostered a culture of creativity within her agency. By encouraging her team members to embrace their unique working styles, Sarah created an agile, dynamic team where hyperfocus could thrive, ultimately driving innovation and growth.

Channeling Hyperfocus: Practical Strategies

To leverage hyperfocus effectively, individuals with ADHD can implement several strategies. Understanding that hyperfocus often arises in response to passion is critical. Here are a few ways to channel this superpower:

1. **Identify Interest Areas**: Understanding what truly captivates their attention can help individuals prioritize projects and commitments that will likely spark hyperfocus.
2. **Create an Environment that Minimizes Distractions**: Individuals should consider developing a workspace that limits interruptions. This may involve noise-canceling headphones or dedicated time slots for deep work.
3. **Set Time Blocks**: By establishing short, focused periods (e.g., using the Pomodoro Technique), individuals can intentionally engage in hyper-focused work sessions, followed by scheduled breaks.
4. **Establish Clear Goals**: Outlining specific, measurable objectives can help provide direction and clarity, making it easier to enter a state of hyperfocus.
5. **Embrace Passion Projects**: Encouraging engagement in passion-driven projects can naturally trigger hyperfocus. Individuals should strive to find areas of work or hobbies that spark joy and excitement.

The Dual Edge of Hyperfocus

While hyperfocus can lead to incredible achievements, it is essential to acknowledge its dual nature. The continued immersion in one task can lead to neglect in other responsibilities or present barriers to maintaining relationships. For example, individuals may miss out on social engagements or neglect daily tasks in favor of prolonged work sessions. Understanding this requires a balance—recognizing when to harness hyperfocus versus when to step back and attend to holistic well-being.

In managing hyperfocus, Alex shares a particular lesson he learned: "I had to become my own project manager. I set alarms to remind myself to take breaks, step outside, and check in with friends. It took practice, but now I can enjoy my work without losing everything else."

Conclusion: Hyperfocus as a Tool for Growth

In celebrating hyperfocus as a trait of ADHD, we approach it as a superpower rather than a limitation. The key is learning to harness it effectively, allowing it to serve as a tool for creativity, innovation, and exceptional achievement. As more individuals like Alex and Sarah share their experiences, the landscape of ADHD continues to shift from negative to positive, emphasizing the extraordinary capabilities that come from understanding and embracing one's unique neurological makeup.

As we explore the multifaceted nature of ADHD in subsequent chapters, remember the stories of those who have channeled hyperfocus into avenues of success. This acknowledgment of ADHD's superpowers is not only liberating but transformative, paving the way for a brighter future for those who dare to embrace their differences.

6

Resilience and Grit: Navigating Challenges

Resilience and grit are often hailed as critical components for success in any endeavor, but for individuals with Attention Deficit Hyperactivity Disorder (ADHD), these traits are not just advantageous—they are often essential. The daily experiences of navigating a world that frequently misinterprets their unique cognitive patterns require a level of perseverance that can only be developed through the challenges they face. In this chapter, we explore how individuals with ADHD cultivate resilience and grit, transforming potential pitfalls into platforms for achievement.

The Foundation of Resilience

At the heart of resilience lies an understanding of adversity as a transformative force. For many living with ADHD, daily challenges—such as difficulties focusing, managing time, and maintaining organization—can seem overwhelming. Yet, these challenges can serve as potent catalysts for personal growth. Each hurdle offers a chance to adapt, develop new strategies, and emerge stronger.

Consider Sarah, a professional athlete whose journey epitomizes the transformative power of resilience. Diagnosed with ADHD at a young age, Sarah constantly felt the pressure to perform at a high level while grappling with impulsivity and distractibility. Instead of viewing her ADHD as an obstacle, she began to see it as part of her unique identity. "I have to work harder than others to channel my energy positively and that has made me incredibly resilient," she explains.

Sarah's journey wasn't without its setbacks. She struggled with inconsistent performance, often losing focus during crucial moments in competitions. Rather than succumbing to frustration, Sarah sought support from coaches and sports psychologists who taught her techniques to manage her symptoms. She installed routines that embedded mindfulness practices, which allowed her to center herself amidst chaos. This willingness to seek help and adapt her training led her to unprecedented levels of success in her sport, including participation in national championships.

The Importance of Grit

While resilience speaks to the ability to bounce back from setbacks, grit encompasses the passion and persistence needed to pursue long-term goals. Individuals with ADHD often exhibit a form of grit fueled by the intense interests and passions they develop. When something captures their attention, their dedication can be unparalleled, paving the way for extraordinary achievements.

Take the case of Kevin, a software engineer who faced significant challenges with time management and focus. During a particularly tough project, his ADHD prompted overwhelming procrastination and self-doubt. Realizing he needed to change his approach, he narrowed his focus, embracing a project he was genuinely passionate about: developing a mental health app tailored for individuals with ADHD.

Kevin immersed himself in the coding and design elements of the app, harnessing his intense passion to propel him through the roadblocks. His fascination with user experience drove him to conduct extensive interviews, gathering insights from potential users to ensure the app met their needs. This commitment to understanding his audience, combined with his technical skills, culminated in the successful launch of an app that resonated with many who shared similar experiences. Kevin's grit not only led to personal satisfaction but also provided a valuable tool for others navigating their mental health journeys.

The Research Behind Resilience

Research supports the notion that individuals with ADHD often develop unique coping strategies that enhance their resilience. A study conducted at the University of California, Berkeley, highlighted that young adults with ADHD demonstrated a stronger capacity for adaptive coping mechanisms compared to their peers without ADHD. This heightened ability to navigate challenges enables individuals with ADHD to constructively manage their difficulties and emerge with a deeper understanding of themselves.

The study also indicated that individuals with ADHD often develop robust problem-solving skills—an attribute closely linked to resilience. When confronted with obstacles, their creative ways of thinking encourage diverse solutions. They learn to reframe their challenges positively, instilling a belief that they can overcome and achieve their goals.

In the following sections, we will delve deeper into specific coping strategies individuals with ADHD have adopted, drawing upon the insights of both research and personal testimonials.

Unique Coping Strategies

One such strategy thriving among individuals with ADHD is the concept of 'reframing.' This involves altering the perspective one takes on a challenge. For instance, when individuals with ADHD struggle to meet a deadline, they may perceive it as a reflection of their inadequacy. However, reframing allows them to recognize it as an opportunity for innovative solutions—developing systems that actively engage their strengths.

Jennifer, a marketing executive, faced this challenge consistently. "I would often find myself racing against the clock, but when I changed how I viewed those moments—from stressors to challenges that fueled my creativity—I became more productive," she shared. Jennifer learned to embrace her spontaneous nature He began scouting locations to work in novel environments, which invigorated her creative process and helped stave off the anxiety related to looming deadlines.

Another prevalent strategy is harnessing the power of community. Connecting with others who share similar experiences serves as a robust support system, reinforcing an individual's sense of belonging. Online forums, support groups, or ADHD communities offer safe spaces for individuals to share their challenges and triumphs. This communal approach fosters resilience as collective experiences create a profound sense of empowerment.

Consider the case of Matt, a young entrepreneur with ADHD who established an online platform for networking among ADHD professionals. "Through my struggles, I realized the strength found in community," he reflected. Matt's initiative allowed him and others to share coping strategies, challenges, and successes, reinforcing a belief that together they could navigate the complexities of ADHD with greater ease.

Emphasizing the Learning Process

A core element of resilience in ADHD is the understanding that failure does not equate to defeat. Embracing a learning mindset allows individuals to perceive setbacks as stepping stones rather than barriers. Jennifer's earlier reflection illustrates this: "Every missed opportunity taught me something invaluable. I learned to adjust my strategies continually, whether it was revising my timeline or incorporating breaks into my workflow." This willingness to adapt fosters a profound resilience, as each challenge serves to sharpen their skills and self-awareness.

A study published in the Journal of Attention Disorders highlighted that individuals with ADHD who cultivated a growth mindset—viewing their abilities as malleable rather than fixed—showed increased resilience and less anxiety regarding performance.

Conclusion: Resilience as a Superpower

Ultimately, resilience and grit are not merely strategies for coping with ADHD; they represent a unique superpower that individuals can harness to navigate life's complexities. By embracing their challenges rather than resisting them, people with ADHD develop a toolkit filled with creative problem-solving skills, adaptability, and community support—all crucial elements for personal and professional success.

As we've seen throughout this chapter, resilience cultivated through the lens of ADHD allows individuals to transmute their experiences into strengths, propelling them forward in ways they may have never anticipated. The journey may be fraught with obstacles, but in recognizing the power they hold, individuals with ADHD are equipped to unleash the superpower within themselves, leading to a life full of potential and promise.

7

Social Skills and Innovation: The Connector's Edge

In a world that often prizes sameness, individuals with Attention Deficit Hyperactivity Disorder (ADHD) stand out not just for their energy or propensity for creativity but for their remarkable ability to connect with others. This chapter delves into the unique social skills and empathetic qualities often exhibited by those with ADHD, highlighting how these traits translate into powerful advantages in personal and professional spheres. Through anecdotes and case studies, we will explore how these connectors harness their innate abilities, leading to innovation and collaboration.

The Essence of Connection

To understand the connector's edge, one must first recognize the nature of social interactions for individuals with ADHD. Far from being socially impaired, many with ADHD display vibrant social skills. Their propensity toward hyperactivity often translates into an engaging demeanor, making them approachable and charismatic. This charm frequently creates an opportunity for establishing connections, allowing them to network effortlessly.

Consider the story of Olivia, a community leader in her city. Olivia was diagnosed with ADHD at a young age and often struggled in traditional environments due to her impulsivity and fidgeting. However, she found solace and empowerment in community service. "When I'm helping people, I feel alive," she says. Her ADHD provided her with an uncanny ability to connect deeply with others, often empathizing with their struggles on a visceral level.

In her role as a community leader, Olivia orchestrated initiatives that required collaboration with city officials, local businesses, and community members. "It's like I can see the needs of others when we're in a room together. I feel a magnetic pull toward addressing their concerns," she explains. Olivia's ADHD gives her a unique perspective, allowing her to foster relationships that bridge gaps and create bridges in her community.

Empathy as a Catalyst for Innovation

Empathy is one of the hallmarks of ADHD, enabling individuals to understand and relate to a wide array of experiences. This capacity for emotional understanding facilitates a deeper awareness of the needs and motivations of others, fostering collaboration and innovation. When these qualities are harnessed, they can lead to significant societal advancements.

Take the case of David, a tech entrepreneur known for his unconventional approach to product development. Diagnosed with ADHD in his early twenties, he found that his challenges in focusing became a superpower when channeled into understanding users' needs. "I often jump around with my ideas, but

I always come back to people. What do they want? What will make their lives easier?" he recounts.

David used his social intuition to build an inclusive team environment, encouraging diverse inputs and ideas. As a result, his startup launched a product that not only addressed a gap in the market but resonated deeply with users on an emotional level. The team was united not just by their skills but by a shared understanding forged by David's ability to empathize and innovate based on the collective experiences of their audience.

Building Networks and Fostering Collaboration

Effective networking is another area where individuals with ADHD often excel. This is particularly true in entrepreneurial and leadership roles, where collaboration and connection can become the bedrock of business success. The dynamic nature of ADHD—characterized by quick thinking and adaptability—often leads to the forging of partnerships that result in innovative projects.

Consider the case of Nour, a vibrant young woman who founded a non-profit organization aimed at promoting mental health awareness. She admits that her ADHD made her journey bumpy; from forgetting scheduled meetings to struggling with organization. Nevertheless, it was her passion and intuitive social skills that enabled her to connect with various stakeholders in her community, including schools, health organizations, and local artists.

"I have a million thoughts flying in my head, and at times, I can't keep track of everything," Nour shares. "But when I meet someone who resonates with my mission, it feels electric. It drives me to share my vision and get them involved, and that's when magic happens." Nour's ADHD, characterized by impulsivity and high energy, pushed her to form alliances with individuals who care deeply about mental health, leading to community-wide initiatives.

Beyond that, her empathetic nature cultivated a safe space for dialogues about mental health, prompting schools to adopt programs addressing the needs of students facing similar challenges. The connections she built did not just spur her organization's growth; they inspired an entire community.

The Science Behind Social Skills in ADHD

Looking at the neuroscience behind ADHD offers insights into why individuals with ADHD are often so social and empathetic. Research indicates that areas of the brain associated with social cognition, such as the medial prefrontal cortex, may function differently in individuals with ADHD. This may heighten their ability to read social cues and express emotions. These neural mechanisms allow individuals to engage dynamically with those around them, and to adapt their communications to different audiences.

Moreover, studies have shown that the dopamine system, which plays a critical role in motivation and reward processing, is often hyperactive in individuals with ADHD. This heightened sensitivity can amplify social experiences, creating a deep-seated motivation to engage with others, share ideas, and lead teams, as these interactions can enhance feelings of achievement.

Fostering an Environment for Connection

Recognizing the social strengths of individuals with ADHD invites a broader discussion about cultivating environments that support such connections. Whether in schools, workplaces, or community settings, there is a growing realization that embracing neurodiversity can lead to richer and more innovative experiences for all involved.

Educators and employers can play a pivotal role in this. By providing platforms for individuals with ADHD to express their social skills, they can facilitate stronger teams, more vibrant communities, and innovative solutions to complex problems. For example, creating collaborative projects that emphasize teamwork and interpersonal interactions can help those with ADHD thrive and capitalize on their strengths.

Conclusion: Embracing the Connector's Edge

As we reflect on the connector's edge provided by ADHD, it is essential to celebrate the empathy, social skills, and collaborative spirit that many individuals with ADHD possess. Their ability to forge relationships and unite diverse voices is not merely a byproduct of their condition; it is a powerful superpower.

In a world that can often feel disconnected, recognizing and harnessing these traits has the potential to fuel innovation and community growth. By cherishing and advocating for the social strengths of individuals with ADHD, we pave the way for a more inclusive society where everyone can find their voice, contribute their ideas, and, ultimately, thrive together.

8

Finding Your Passion: The Key to Motivation

In the vast landscape of human endeavor, motivation acts as the compass needle guiding individuals toward their true north—their passions. For many with Attention Deficit Hyperactivity Disorder (ADHD), finding and tapping into these passions is not merely a beneficial pursuit; it is often a necessity. When ADHD manifests, it can sometimes overshadow interest and engagement, transforming potential focus into a struggle against distractions. Yet, when individuals with ADHD align their pursuits with their passions, transformative experiences often unfold.

Finding passion serves as a fundamental building block for success, self-fulfillment, and overall well-being. It is an exhilarating journey that leads one to their most authentic self while simultaneously framing their distinctive ADHD attributes in a new light—an empowering force that propels them forward. In this chapter, we will explore the dynamics of motivation and passion for those with ADHD through the lens of individuals who have successfully converted their hobbies and interests into thriving careers.

The Joy of Discovery: An Author's Journey

Consider the journey of Julia, an author and a dreamer, whose ADHD has often felt like a double-edged sword. The world around her was full of noise—constructively chaotic, yet frequently overwhelming. As a child, Julia was intrigued by the imaginative worlds crafted within the pages of her favorite books, but her struggle with attentional focus often left her feeling incapable of achieving the same creativity.

One day, while emptying her closet, she stumbled upon an old journal filled with short stories penned as a teenager. As she read through her youthful words, she felt a surge of nostalgia and an unexpected flicker of joy. At that moment, fueled by an instinctively understanding friend's encouragement, she resolved to publish her work. Writing became her conduit—an arena where her imagination ran wild, her hyperactive brain transformed into a productive engine, and her heart found solace.

Julia's passion for storytelling reshaped her experience with ADHD. Once perceived as a barrier, it became a tool for expressing the vivid imagination that her ADHD had fostered. It wasn't the structured writing process that drove her; instead, it was the unfettered exploration of her ideas, characters, and settings that lit her creative flame. The process served as both an escape and a method, allowing her brain to explore without bounds. When writing, Julia tapped into her hyperfocus; hours could slip by as she transformed her thoughts into vibrant narratives.

As her stories gained traction and resonance among readers, Julia discovered the importance of passion in fueling her motivation. The act of writing became a transformative experience.

With every completed manuscript, she healed her relationship with ADHD, no longer viewing it as a hindrance but as an empowering ally in her creative journey.

Real-World Transformations: Hobbies to Ventures

Julia's journey represents a broader theme where countless individuals with ADHD have discovered the powerful link between passionate pursuits and sustained motivation—in both big and small dreams. When passions are pursued, mundane tasks can morph into stimulating challenges, and barriers that once felt insurmountable begin to shift.

John, a former marketing professional and now a full-time chef, uncovered his passion through a community cooking class. The zest and excitement of culinary creativity were palpable—a stark contrast to the bland, routine tasks of his desk job. Inspired by cooking shows and driven by his desire to innovate, John dove into the world of gastronomy. The colorful goodies dancing around him in the kitchen stimulated his senses beyond what months of endless spreadsheets ever offered.

As he honed his culinary techniques, the hyperfocus of ADHD propelled him to develop his own unique recipes, blending flavors and techniques into stunning dishes that received praise from friends and family. With burning excitement, he began sharing his culinary adventures on social media, attracting a community of food enthusiasts along the way. Soon recognized for his knack for presentation and flavor, John transformed his passion into a thriving catering business.

For individuals like John and Julia, passion-driven pursuits have unveiled a profound understanding of their ADHD traits. The challenges once associated with their conditions—restlessness, distraction, and impulsivity—became the very qualities that forged their pathways to entrepreneurial success.

The Science of Passion and Motivation in ADHD

Research supports the transformational role of passion in elevating motivation, particularly for individuals with ADHD. Studies show that intrinsic motivation—driven by personal interests—leads to enhanced engagement and success in both academic and professional settings. When individuals immerse themselves in activities that resonate with their passions, they bypass the difficulties associated with distractions and impulsivity, liberating their energy towards productive outputs.

An extensive study highlighted how individuals with ADHD, when working within their areas of passion, demonstrated improved focus, resilience, and creative problem-solving abilities. The neural pathways that govern attention and reward processing in the brain are more actively engaged, fostering an environment ripe for innovation and clarity.

For many, the journey to discover their passions is surreal and evolving. It serves as a process of exploration that may require patience, introspection, and openness to new experiences. Like Julia's and John's stories, success often thrives on ambition, enthusiasm, and heart-driven pursuits.

Cultivating Passion: Practical Strategies

To ensure individuals with ADHD find their passions, several strategies can be employed:

1. **Explore Diverse Interests**: Encourage experimentation with various hobbies and activities to uncover latent passions. From painting and photography to cooking and technology, diversity is key.

2. **Set Flexible Goals**: Instead of overwhelming oneself with rigid structures, create fluid, short-term goals to keep enthusiasm alive. Acknowledge the evolving nature of passions.
3. **Connect with Like-minded Communities**: Seeking out others who share similar interests fosters both inspiration and motivation. Oftentimes, community interaction can spark a new passion.
4. **Embrace Change**: Passions can shift over time. Be open to change and adaptable in pursuing new avenues, as many individuals find fresh areas of interest awaken later in life.
5. **Integrate Passion with Responsibilities**: Infuse daily responsibilities with aspects of identified passions. For instance, if someone loves writing, maintaining a blog or journaling can add creativity to routine tasks.

Conclusion: The Empowering Journey Ahead

Finding one's passion is an introspective journey that fuels both identity and motivation—a noteworthy endeavor, especially for individuals with ADHD. The stories of individuals like Julia and John have illustrated not just the possibility of success but the assurance that passion can interlace with ADHD traits to cultivate a superpower of its own.

As we celebrate the myriad gifts within this community, it becomes essential to encourage recognition of personal passions. When individuals with ADHD align their pursuits with genuine interests, they illuminate their paths with boundless energy, creativity, and spirit. This journey is not merely about finding interests; it's about embracing the adventure, unlocking motivation, and recognizing that the greatest joys often bloom from the passions that reflect our authentic selves.

In future chapters, we will explore practical tools, strategies, and success stories that empower readers not just to recognize their passions but to cultivate them into sustainable practices that enrich their lives profoundly. Let the journey to passion, motivation, and the acknowledgment of the ADHD superpower continue to unfold with exuberance and excitement.

9

Tools for Transformation: Practical Strategies for Harnessing ADHD

In today's fast-paced world, many individuals with Attentional Deficit Hyperactivity Disorder (ADHD) often find themselves struggling to keep pace. Despite the overwhelming challenges, this chapter focuses on practical tools and strategies that can effectively harness the unique traits associated with ADHD and channel them into productive avenues. By equipping individuals with specific techniques and modifications, we can turn potential obstacles into notable strengths.

Understanding the Landscape: The Need for Transformation

For decades, ADHD has been framed through a lens of disorder and dysfunction, leaving many wondering how to reconcile their struggles with a desire to lead fulfilling lives. However, emerging research suggests that with the right tools and strategies, individuals with ADHD can navigate challenges skillfully, turning their neurodivergent wiring into powerful motivators. The right modifications, whether at home, in school, or in the workplace, can significantly influence the trajectory of an ADHD individual's life, cultivating resilience, creativity, and ingenuity.

Practical Strategies: Framework for Success

1. **Environment Tailoring**: One of the most effective ways to harness ADHD traits is by modifying one's environment. A middle school teacher named Ms. Rivera demonstrates the impact of creating ADHD-friendly classrooms. After observing her students grapple with standard classroom setups that often provoked distractions, she decided to transform her teaching strategies. She incorporated various seating options—like standing desks, bean bags, and fidget tools.

Anecdote: "I noticed my students thrived when they had a choice," Ms. Rivera recalls. "When given the option to stand or sit, they engaged more actively with the material. I even incorporated 'brain breaks' where students could choose short, physical activities. The difference was palpable—they were more focused during instruction and excelled during assessments!" By aligning the physical space with the students' needs, she empowered them to take charge of their learning journey.

1. **Time Management Techniques**: For many individuals with ADHD, time can feel elastic, often stretching or compressing in ways that disrupt productivity. Utilizing timers, apps, or visual scheduling tools can serve as game-changers.

Case Study: Consider Jason, a software developer with ADHD. He struggled immensely with project deadlines until he discovered the Pomodoro Technique—an approach advocating for 25 minutes of focused work followed by a 5-minute break. "I found it changed how I approached my tasks," Jason shares. "I could hyper-focus within the 25 minutes and would reward myself with a break, which prepared me for the next sprint." Such strategies can help individuals navigate the often daunting task of time management more effectively.

1. **Setting Goals with Clarity**: Goals can be daunting, particularly for someone with ADHD, where the allure of novelty often leads to shiny-object syndrome. Instead of overwhelming oneself with multiple objectives, setting Specific, Measurable, Achievable, Relevant, and Time-bound (SMART) goals is vital.

Anecdote: Emma, an aspiring writer with ADHD, faced constant frustration as she juggled half-finished manuscripts. With the guidance of a mentor, she learned to establish SMART goals for her writing career. "Focusing on one project at a time transformed my writing," Emma reflects. "Instead of saying, 'I'll finish my book,' I told myself, 'I'll complete five pages by Friday.' Breaking it down made it feel doable and less intimidating."

1. **Utilizing Technology**: Technology offers a plethora of tools designed to enhance organization, promote concentration, and structure daily activities. From project management tools like Trello or Asana to calendar apps that promote reminders, the options are endless.

Case Study: A startup founded by an entrepreneur with ADHD utilized technology to foster a productive work environment. They implemented software that not only manages tasks but also allows the team to visually track their progress. The result? Employees reported feeling less overwhelmed and more focused, noting that the accountability offered by these tools nurtured collaboration and transparency.

1. **Incorporation of Mindfulness and Physical Activity**: Physical activity and mindfulness practices have gained recognition for their capabilities to regulate attention and improve focus. Brief, intentional breaks—like a 10-minute walk or a short meditation—can serve as effective resets.

Anecdote: John, an athlete with ADHD, found success in his career by incorporating mindfulness tactics before major competitions. "I started using visualization techniques to prepare for races. Taking time to breathe and focus kept my nerves in check," he explains. The practice not only prepared him mentally but also boosted his performance.

1. **Building a Support Network**: No journey is undertaken alone, and having a robust support network is imperative for success. Communities—whether they are friends, family, or professional organizations—can instill motivation, accountability, and understanding.

Case Study: Meet Sylvia, who faced intense insecurity due to her ADHD in a corporate setting. She formed a support group within her workplace, where individuals shared their experiences, ideas, and coping strategies. "What surprised me was how many people in high-pressure roles felt the same way I did," Sylvia reflects. The group not only fostered dialogue but also led to the implementation of ADHD-friendly policies within the organization.

Embracing the Unique Journey of ADHD

As we think about effective strategies for harnessing the strengths of ADHD, it is vital to remember that each individual's journey is unique. What works for one person may not for another; thus, flexibility and individuality are essential components of the process.

Moreover, the transformation from perceived disorder to celebrated strengths requires a collective effort. There must be a cultural shift—encompassing schools, workplaces, and communities—where ADHD is viewed more as a superpower than a hindrance. Education and awareness initiatives can educate those around us, promoting understanding and reducing stigma, which has historically surrounded ADHD.

Conclusion: Creating a Toolkit for Success

The tools and techniques outlined in this chapter represent just a glimpse into the myriad strategies available to unleash the superpowers of ADHD. By refocusing on strengths rather than weaknesses and approaching challenges with innovation and creativity, individuals with ADHD can pave the path toward empowerment and success.

As we champion transformation and adaptability, our narrative around ADHD can evolve. Building environments that empower individuals with ADHD to thrive is not merely an option—it's an obligation. With the right tools, we can collectively transform lives, elevating the message that ADHD is not merely a condition to manage, but a unique tapestry of strengths ready to be celebrated.

10

Education: Changing the Narrative in Schools

In the journey of recognizing ADHD not just as a challenge but as an inherent superpower, the educational system plays a critical role. For too long, schools operated under outdated assumptions that ADHD was merely a behavioral disorder needing remedy through strict discipline or medication. However, an evolving paradigm has emerged—one that embraces the unique qualities of students with ADHD, enabling them to thrive. This chapter delves into the transformative changes occurring in educational environments, highlighting how tailored approaches cater to the strengths of ADHD students.

The Need for Change

The traditional classroom often mirrors a factory assembly line. Students are expected to fit into uniform molds—sitting quietly, maintaining focus for extended periods, and absorbing information in a linear fashion. For students with ADHD, these expectations can often feel suffocating. Imagine being asked to sit still for hours, with a mind that dances rapidly through thoughts, ideas, and possibilities. The conventional approach, while well-intentioned, risks stifling the very creativity and innovation that students with ADHD possess.

But change is on the horizon. More awareness about the strengths and unique traits associated with ADHD has prompted educators and policy-makers to rethink classroom dynamics. Schools are beginning to adopt personalized learning models, recognizing that each student's unique challenges can also herald boundless potential.

A Student's Story: Embracing Individuality

Sarah was just another kid in a large crowd of middle school students battling the chaos of adolescence. Diagnosed with ADHD, she frequently found herself in trouble for daydreaming instead of paying attention in class. Labelled as a troublemaker, she struggled to see herself as anything more than a misfit in a system that valued conformity over creativity. Her report cards bore evidence of her struggle: "Could do better if she paid attention," read the comments, a refrain familiar to many ADHD students.

Yet one day, everything changed when a new teacher, Mr. Johnson, arrived at her school. Mr. Johnson had experience in working with students diagnosed with ADHD, and his first act of change was to break the conventional mold. Instead of viewing Sarah through a deficit lens, he recognized her lively imagination and boundless energy as potential assets.

Mr. Johnson introduced an interactive learning environment

where movement was encouraged. He transformed his classroom into a dynamic space filled with art supplies, interactive whiteboards, and flexible seating options. Most importantly, he voiced his understanding that ADHD was not an impediment but a different lens through which Sarah viewed the world.

"Math made no sense, but can I draw it?" Sarah asked, her eyes brightening as she walked over to a large whiteboard.

"Absolutely," Mr. Johnson replied, clearly thrilled by her initiative.

Sarah blossomed under this new regime. Her engagement soared, and her test scores began reflecting the girl she knew she could be. Instead of rote answers, her assessment projects displayed intricate connections, surprising insights, and creative problem-solving approaches. The experience was not just a personal victory; it was a confirmation of the need for educational reform—validation for her unique mind.

Modern Educational Approaches

The transformative story of Sarah isn't an isolated incident but rather emblematic of a growing trend in education to accommodate ADHD students' strengths. Programs focused on personalized learning, project-based education, and social-emotional learning are becoming increasingly popular.

The Implementation of Tailored Programs

Schools are recognizing that the one-size-fits-all model is ineffective. Programs tailored specifically for ADHD students often incorporate a range of strategies that emphasize engagement, creativity, and motivation. For example, a project-based learning approach allows students to immerse themselves actively in their studies. Knowledge is acquired not through passive reception but through exploration and real-world application, tapping into the inherent curiosity of ADHD students.

Moreover, schools are introducing teacher training programs focused on neurodiversity. Educators learn to appreciate the unique skill sets of students with ADHD—not merely how to manage their behaviors but how to empower them. This pedagogical shift emphasizes understanding the neurological underpinnings of ADHD, helping teachers to connect better with their students.

Case Study: An Innovative School Program

Consider Greenfield Academy, a school that implemented a program specifically designed for students with ADHD. The initiative comprises small class sizes, varied teaching methods, and a flexible daily schedule. Students attend core classes but engage in "Innovation Labs"—interactive sessions where they can explore interests ranging from robotics to creative writing.

A research partnership with a local university assessed the program's impact. Results came back profound: students' academic performance rose significantly, attendance improved, and disciplinary issues dropped sharply. Beyond statistics, students reported feeling more empowered and engaged in their learning, with many expressing newfound clarity about their futures.

An illustrative moment came from a student's project in the Innovation Lab. Alex, an 11-year-old boy with ADHD, was passionate about technology. He decided to build a simple app to help students with ADHD track their assignments and manage their time more effectively. Under the mentorship of enthusiastic teachers and support staff, Alex dedicated his hyperfocus to this project, working late into the evenings. His app prototype ultimately won recognition at a regional tech fair, symbolizing the impact of an education system that nurtured rather than stifled.

Rethinking Evaluation Methods

Assessment methods are also evolving. Traditional grading structures often fail to encapsulate the unique contributions and thoughts of ADHD students. Schools are considering project-based evaluations, peer reviews, and portfolios that allow students to showcase their understanding creatively. These methods permit ADHD students to demonstrate knowledge without the constraints of a conventional testing environment, leading to more accurate appraisals of their abilities and interests.

Sarah's story again highlights this shift. She was no longer defined by her ability to sit still and regurgitate facts but rather by her creativity and innovative ideas, elements that could flourish within the supportive and tailored educational framework provided by Mr. Johnson's approach.

The Road Ahead

The narrative surrounding ADHD in educational institutions is undeniably shifting. As society begins to appreciate the potential inherent within ADHD individuals, schools are becoming bastions for positive change—environments that welcome diversity in cognitive processing and learning styles. As seen through the lens of personal stories and supported by research, students are not merely surviving; they are flourishing, achieving academic and personal milestones that were once thought unreachable.

As we move forward, the challenge remains to sustain and expand these changes across educational systems worldwide. It calls upon teachers, administrators, and parents to advocate for ADHD awareness, ensuring every child can unleash their superpowers in a nurturing, accepting environment.

Change is indeed on the horizon, and it is crucial to foster an educational narrative that champions the strengths of students with ADHD—transformative powerhouses capable of changing not only their own futures but also the world around them.

11

In the Workplace: Transforming Career Paths

In today's dynamic economy, where creativity, adaptability, and rapid innovation are paramount, it is becoming increasingly evident that traditional perspectives of work must evolve. In this transformational landscape, those diagnosed with Attention Deficit Hyperactivity Disorder (ADHD) stand out, often showcasing unique skills that can be harnessed to advance not just their careers but also the organizations they are part of. This chapter delves into how to leverage ADHD traits in the workplace for professional growth and satisfaction.

The Unseen Value of ADHD

For far too long, ADHD has been misunderstood and misrepresented as a mere disorder—a set of challenges that hinder professional performance and success. However, an increasing number of professionals and organizations are beginning to recognize ADHD as a platform for innovative thinking and problem-solving. The unique wiring of an ADHD brain often leads to insights that others may overlook or dismiss. This reframing gives hope and guidance to both individuals with ADHD and the employers who aim to nurture their latent strengths.

One individual who successfully navigated this terrain is Olivia, a corporate leader at a tech startup. Olivia vividly recalls the challenges she faced early in her career. The conventional work environment was a minefield of distractions and rigidity that stifled her creativity. Yet, she discovered that her ADHD-informed approach led her to develop unconventional yet effective solutions in high-pressure situations. "I remember staring at a complex problem—most people would have taken a long time to dissect it," she shares. "But I could see it in my mind like a puzzle. My brain was already imagining multiple angles and possibilities."

Her story exemplifies the potential for remarkable achievement when ADHD traits are embraced rather than suppressed. But how do we transform the workplace to enable such empowerment?

Building Environments of Neurodiversity

Organizations that consciously design their workspaces to accommodate neurodiversity are reaping the rewards of their investments. Employing proactive strategies can make a significant difference. For instance, companies like Microsoft and Siemens have established neurodiversity hiring programs. These initiatives focus on creating roles tailored to individual strengths, facilitating environments where creativity can flourish.

A fascinating case study comes from SAP, a multinational enterprise applications company that launched the "Autism at Work" program. This initiative was designed to recruit individuals on the autism spectrum while also being inclusive of those with ADHD. The results were encouraging; not only did the initiative foster innovation, but it also led to an increase in overall team performance. Employees reported feeling more engaged, knowing their unique contributions were valued.

Mary, a participant in the program, recounts her experience, stating, "I felt seen for the first time in a work environment. They embraced my differences rather than expected me to fit a mold. The creative problem-solving I brought to the team was my superpower." The success of such initiatives illustrates that organizations committed to neurodiversity not only uplift their employees with ADHD but benefit from the innovative thinking these individuals bring to the table.

Practical Strategies for Individuals with ADHD

It is vital for individuals with ADHD to harness their traits effectively within their careers. Below are some practical strategies drawn from both personal anecdotes and proven approaches used in successful companies:

1. **Utilizing Hyperfocus:** As discussed in previous chapters, hyperfocus can be a double-edged sword. When directed towards meaningful tasks, it can lead to exceptional output. It is essential for individuals with ADHD to identify projects they are passionate about and funnel their energy into those endeavors, creating their ideal workspace to capitalize on their unique focus patterns.
2. **Setting Clear Goals:** The whirlwind of ideas and projects can lead to chaos without a clear path. Breaking tasks down into manageable goals can help individuals with ADHD maintain clarity and direction. Regular check-ins with

colleagues can also help create accountability and offer fresh perspectives on projects.
3. **Leveraging Technology:** Numerous productivity tools can assist in managing time and attention. From planners and time-blocking applications to noise-canceling headphones, utilizing technology to create routines tailored to ADHD can significantly enhance work performance.
4. **Communicating Openly:** As daunting as it may seem, discussing ADHD with colleagues can foster understanding and collaboration. Olivia notes, "At first, I was scared to talk about my ADHD, but once I opened up, my teammates began to understand my work style. It helped build a supportive atmosphere." This transparency often cultivates a culture of empathy and teamwork.
5. **Seek Mentorship and Flexible Work Arrangements:** Finding a mentor can offer guidance on navigating challenges within the workplace. Moreover, flexible work arrangements, where individuals can operate on their own terms—be it using remote work options or creating a personalized schedule—enable employees to work at their most productive times.

Transformative Leadership

Leadership also plays a critical role in fostering an ADHD-friendly workplace culture. Leaders who understand the strengths of neurodiverse thinkers can create environments that celebrate innovation. A notable example is David, a CEO at an established marketing agency who himself has ADHD. He emphasizes hiring individuals with diverse neurological backgrounds, as they provide different perspectives to the team.

"In my experience, the best ideas often come from an unexpected angle," David asserts. "Those with ADHD challenge conventional thinking, they don't just solve problems—they redefine how we see them."

His leadership approach is about dismantling stigma, providing mentorship, and celebrating the contributions of all employees. By doing so, he ensures that the company not only reaps the benefits of neurodiversity but also fosters a culture of collaboration and creativity that benefits everyone involved.

Career Satisfaction for All

A workplace that recognizes ADHD as a superpower not only promotes individual success but also contributes significantly to overall company health. With the right strategies in place, organizations can witness enhanced creativity, increased problem-solving capacity, and overall satisfaction from employees.

For individuals with ADHD, the workplace becomes a platform for them to rise uniquely and confidently. The superpower no longer stays hidden; it's transformed into a beacon of innovation and productivity. As we move towards a more inclusive future, the recognition and harnessing of neurodiversity will remain essential, providing value not only to individuals but to society as a whole.

In conclusion, ADHD is an invaluable asset in the workplace—a superpower waiting to be unleashed. By embracing these differences and rewiring the traditional expectations surrounding work, we create a flourishing ecosystem that benefits everyone involved. The journey from a misunderstood disorder to a celebrated approach is not only possible; it is already underway. As we step into this new era, let us encourage one another to embrace our unique contributions and redefine what it means to overcome challenges in the workplace.

12

Conclusion: Celebrating the Superpower Within

As we draw the curtains on our exploration into ADHD, it becomes exceedingly clear that it is time we collectively shift our perceptions. Traditionally, ADHD has been viewed through a narrow lens—one that often paints individuals as challenged, distracted, or disordered. Yet, as we have delved deep into the nuances of ADHD, a resounding narrative emerges: this condition is not merely a list of deficits but a canvas of superpowers waiting to be unlocked. Throughout this book, we have uncovered a rich tapestry of strengths and contributions that individuals with ADHD bring to our world—a phenomenon that deserves celebration.

Locking back on the journey, the tone that evolves through personal stories, case studies, and scientific explorations illustrates an inspiring portrait of what it means to live with and around ADHD. Take, for instance, the spirited account of the community of individuals with ADHD who came together in a shared space, amplifying each other's voices. Their self-formed support network met weekly to discuss personal achievements, challenges, and strategies. With a contagious energy, they shared anecdotes like badges of honor; tales of creativity ignited during marathon brainstorming sessions, moments when hyperfocus transformed into extraordinary outcomes, and stories of resilience that highlighted their journeys through the ups and downs of daily life.

One powerful anecdote shared during these gatherings was from a father of a teenager diagnosed with ADHD. He recounted how his son had once struggled immensely in school but, in a serendipitous turn of events, discovered his talent for graphic design through a summer workshop. The captivating freedom of creativity unleashed a passion that translated into excellence, propelling him forward and reminding the group that challenges often give birth to new strengths. The father's pride in his son, who had transformed his "struggle" into a "superpower," resonated deeply among attendees, reaffirming the unyielding spirit that thrives within them.

This journey is not just anecdotal; it is grounded in solid research and studies that reinforce ADHD as a source of innovation, creativity, resilience, and leadership. Indeed, we examined numerous case studies throughout this book, highlighting groundbreaking entrepreneurs, dazzling artists, and visionary leaders who have all utilized their ADHD traits to pivot their lives in remarkable directions. These stories attest to the fact that the greatest contributions to society often arise from those who think differently, approach problems from unique angles, and embrace their own brand of ingenuity.

One such case was that of a tech startup founded by individuals with ADHD, who, through their comprehensive understanding of their unique strengths, developed an application that made waves across the industry. Their approach to brainstorming sessions involved playful engagements that allowed chaotic thoughts to dance freely, leading to out-of-the-box solutions that conventional methodologies simply could not replicate. This not only showcased the immense potential fostering within people with ADHD but also illuminated the importance of creating environments where such talents can be nurtured and harnessed.

As we reflect on our findings, we cannot overlook the importance of community and support systems. The collective voice of individuals with ADHD empowers not just those within the circle but also fosters a broader understanding in society at large. This brings us to a powerful call to action: we must advocate for ADHD awareness, ensuring that individuals are met with empathy, understanding, and opportunities to thrive. Schools, workplaces, and public institutions must continue to evolve, moving away from outdated methods that perceive ADHD solely as a hurdle to be overcome. Instead, they should embrace tailored approaches that recognize ADHD's unique strengths. Each individual contributes something vital and distinct, creating a richer, more diverse tapestry in our communities.

Moreover, we should harness our understanding of ADHD to educate those outside the ADHD community—friends, family, educators, and employers—about the diverse strengths that reside within. An increasing number of companies are beginning to champion neurodiversity, celebrating the unique skills and perspectives of individuals with ADHD. They recognize how these traits drive innovation, enhance teamwork, and propel organizations to new heights. As we move forward, it becomes increasingly imperative that we champion similar initiatives in every facet of society, ensuring that recognition of the superpower within ADHD transforms into tangible support mechanisms for individuals everywhere.

In closing, as we celebrate the superpower within ADHD, let us be relentless in our pursuit of advocacy, inclusion, and understanding. Let us challenge outdated narratives and open our eyes to the boundless possibilities that ADHD can yield. To all the individuals navigating life with ADHD: consider your experiences an unyielding source of strength. Lean into your creativity, embrace your resilience, and allow your hyperfocus to guide you toward your passions. Surround yourself with a community that uplifts and inspires you. Draw strength from one another, and continue to disrupt the conventional landscape with your boundless energy and innovative spirit.

Let this book serve as a reminder that, while ADHD may come with challenges, it also unveils a path to extraordinary opportunities. Celebrate your superpower, share your story, and strive for progress. In doing so, we not only elevate ourselves but also illuminate the way for others who will follow. Together, we can redefine how ADHD is seen—not just as a diagnosis, but as a gateway to a powerful and vibrant future. Here's to the superpowers inherent in each and every one of us, waiting to be unleashed!

www.ingramcontent.com/pod-product-compliance
Lightning Source LLC
Chambersburg PA
CBHW071727020426
42333CB00017B/2421